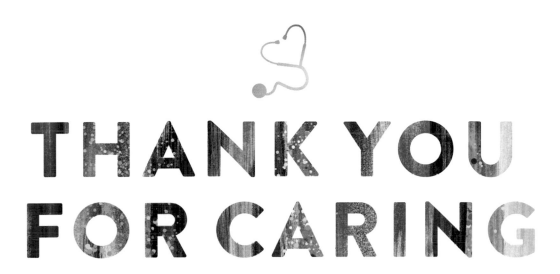

THANK YOU FOR CARING

a celebration of
NURSES, DOCTORS, &
OTHER HEALTH-CARE HEROES

edited by mary zaia

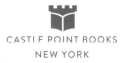

CASTLE POINT BOOKS

NEW YORK

THANK YOU FOR CARING. Copyright © 2020 by St. Martin's Press.
All rights reserved. Printed in Canada. For information,
address St. Martin's Press, 120 Broadway, New York, NY 10271.

www.castlepointbooks.com

The Castle Point Books trademark is owned by Castle Point Publishing, LLC.
Castle Point books are published and distributed by St. Martin's Press.

ISBN 978-1-250-27508-0 (paper over board)
ISBN 978-1-250-27509-7 (ebook)

Design by Tara Long

Images used under license from Shutterstock.com

Our books may be purchased in bulk for promotional, educational, or business use.
Please contact your local bookseller or the Macmillan Corporate and Premium Sales Department
at 1-800-221-7945, extension 5442, or by email at MacmillanSpecialMarkets@macmillan.com.

First Edition: 2020

10 9 8 7 6 5 4 3 2 1

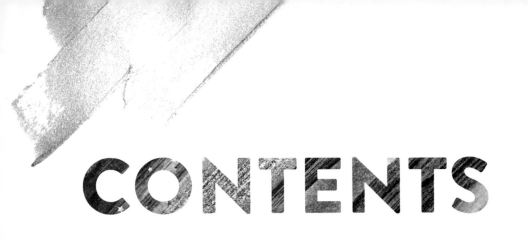

CONTENTS

YOU WERE THERE

FROM FIRST BREATH TO LAST BREATH and for many heart-twisting moments in between, health-care heroes are there, holding hands and soothing souls while providing care. Theirs is a special calling to serve and love people who often walk into their lives as complete strangers. Suddenly, these lives are threaded together by the caregiver's compassion, strength, dedication, and skill. How can we possibly repay the gift of better health, lifted hope, or just comfort in a time of crisis?

Thank You for Caring is a small but powerful way to appreciate the devotion of health-care providers who care for us and our loved ones at some of our most vulnerable times. Each page recognizes the challenging conditions our health-care heroes face so gracefully each day and offers support for all they give to better our world. With this collection of moving quotes, celebrate the extraordinary character of nurses, doctors, and all health-care providers who put others first and touch our lives in so many meaningful ways.

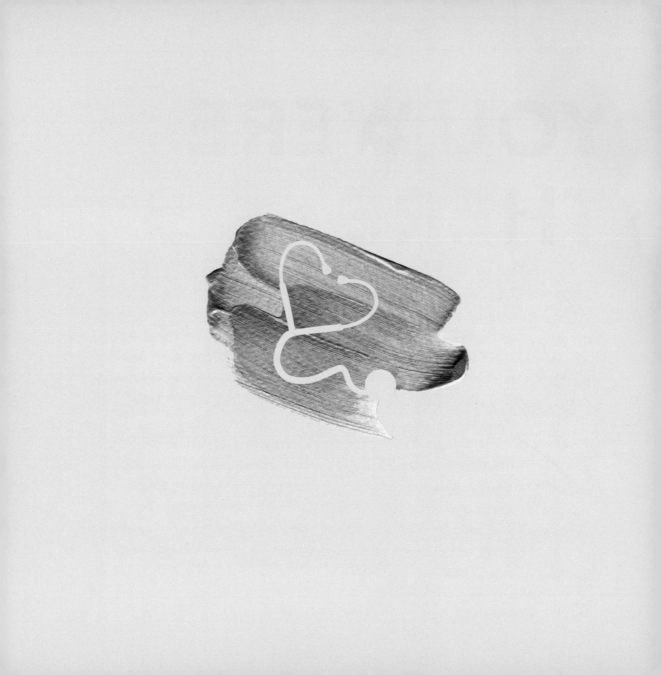

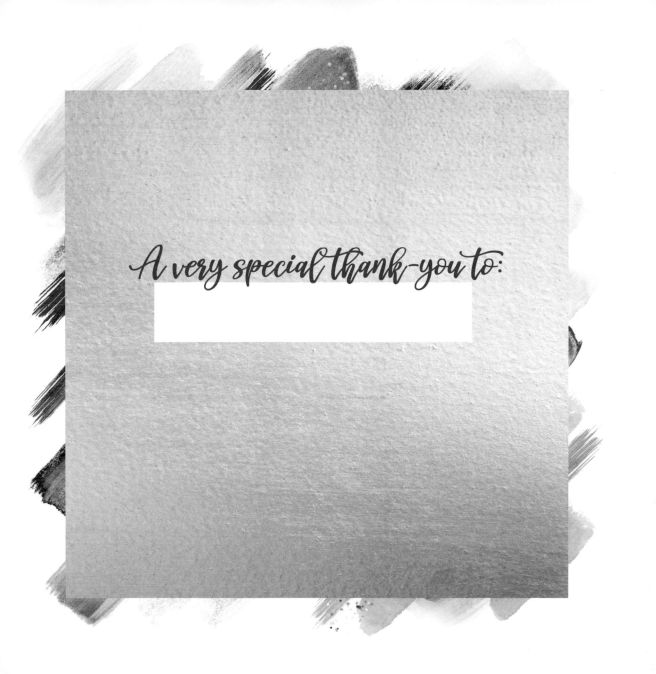

A very special thank-you to:

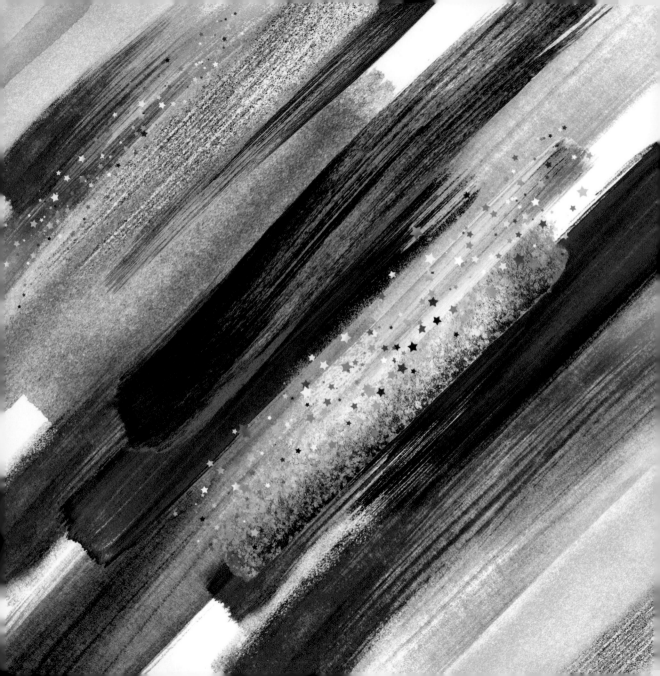

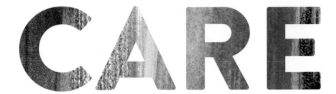
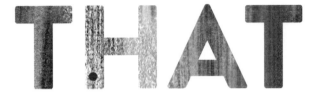
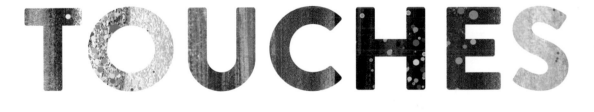
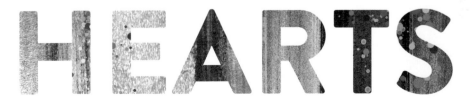

CARE THAT TOUCHES HEARTS

THEY MAY FORGET
YOUR NAME,
BUT THEY WILL
NEVER FORGET
*how you made
them feel.*

MAYA ANGELOU

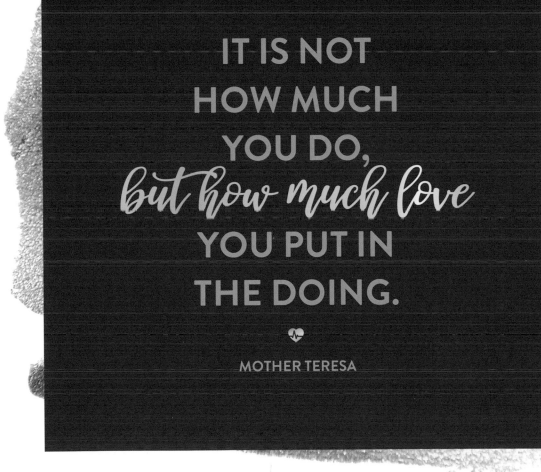

IT IS NOT
HOW MUCH
YOU DO,
but how much love
YOU PUT IN
THE DOING.

MOTHER TERESA

Have a heart
THAT NEVER HARDENS,
a temper
THAT NEVER TIRES,
a touch
THAT NEVER HURTS.

CHARLES DICKENS

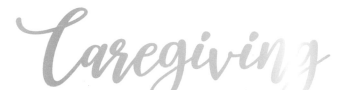

OFTEN CALLS US TO LEAN INTO LOVE WE DIDN'T KNOW POSSIBLE.

TIA WALKER

No book can teach you
HOW TO CRY WITH A PATIENT.
No class can teach you
HOW TO TELL THEIR FAMILY
THAT THEIR PARENTS
HAVE DIED OR ARE DYING.
No professor can teach you
HOW TO FIND DIGNITY IN
GIVING SOMEONE A BED BATH.

It's not about the pills or charting.

IT'S ABOUT
BEING ABLE TO
LOVE PEOPLE WHEN
THEY ARE AT THEIR
WEAKEST MOMENTS.

UNKNOWN

Tenderness and kindness ARE NOT SIGNS OF WEAKNESS AND DESPAIR, BUT MANIFESTATIONS OF *strength and resolution.*

KAHLIL GIBRAN

NURSES DISPENSE
comfort, compassion, and caring
WITHOUT EVEN
A PRESCRIPTION.

VAL SAINTSBURY

WHEN I THINK ABOUT ALL
THE PATIENTS AND THEIR LOVED ONES
I HAVE WORKED WITH OVER THE YEARS,
I KNOW MOST OF THEM
DON'T REMEMBER ME, NOR I THEM.
BUT I DO KNOW THAT I GAVE A LITTLE
PIECE OF MYSELF TO EACH OF THEM,
AND THEY TO ME,
AND THOSE THREADS MAKE UP
THE TAPESTRY THAT IS
MY CAREER IN NURSING.

DONNA WILK CARDILLO

THROUGHOUT HISTORY, *"tender loving care"* HAS UNIFORMLY BEEN RECOGNIZED AS A VALUABLE ELEMENT IN HEALING.

LARRY DOSSEY

PEOPLE PAY THE DOCTOR FOR HIS TROUBLE; *for his kindness* THEY STILL REMAIN IN HIS DEBT.

SENECA

YOU REALLY CAN

change the world

IF YOU

care enough.

♥

MARIAN WRIGHT EDELMAN

Nurse:
JUST ANOTHER WORD
TO DESCRIBE A PERSON
strong enough
TO TOLERATE ANYTHING
and soft enough
TO UNDERSTAND ANYONE.

♡

BRITTANY WILSON

Being deeply loved
BY SOMEONE
GIVES YOU STRENGTH,
while loving
someone deeply
GIVES YOU COURAGE.

LAO TZU

BOUND BY PAPERWORK, SHORT ON HANDS, SLEEP, AND ENERGY...
nurses are rarely short on caring.

♥

SHARON HUDACEK

YOU ARE
goodness and mercy
AND COMPASSION
AND UNDERSTANDING.

NEALE DONALD WALSCH

WE OFTEN THINK OF NURSING
AS GIVING MEDS ON TIME,
CHECKING AN X-RAY TO SEE IF
THE DOCTOR NEEDS TO BE CALLED,
OR TAKING AN ADMISSION AT 2:00 A.M.
WITH A SMILE ON OUR FACE.
TOO OFTEN, WE FORGET
ALL THE OTHER THINGS THAT MAKE
OUR JOB WHAT IT TRULY IS—
*caring and having a desire
to make a difference.*

ERIN PETTENGILL

The capacity to care
IS THE THING
WHICH GIVES LIFE
ITS DEEPEST
SIGNIFICANCE.

PABLO CASALS

WHERE
THERE IS
LOVE
there is
life.

MAHATMA GANDHI

AS A NURSE, WE HAVE
THE OPPORTUNITY
*to heal the heart,
mind, soul, and body*
OF OUR PATIENTS,
THEIR FAMILIES,
AND OURSELVES.

MAYA ANGELOU

Caring is
THE ESSENCE
OF NURSING.

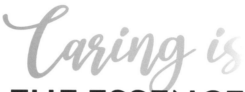

JEAN WATSON

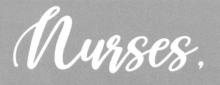

Nurses,
ONE OF THE
FEW BLESSINGS
OF BEING ILL.

SARA MOSS-WOLFE

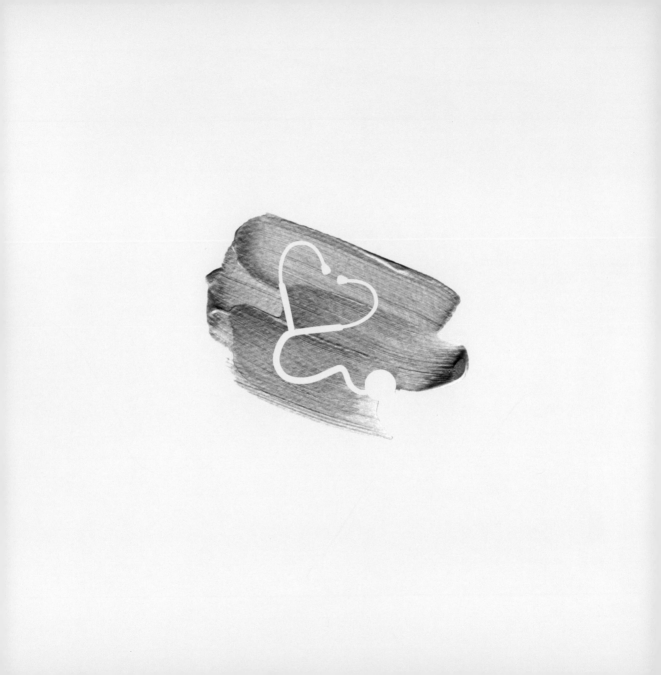

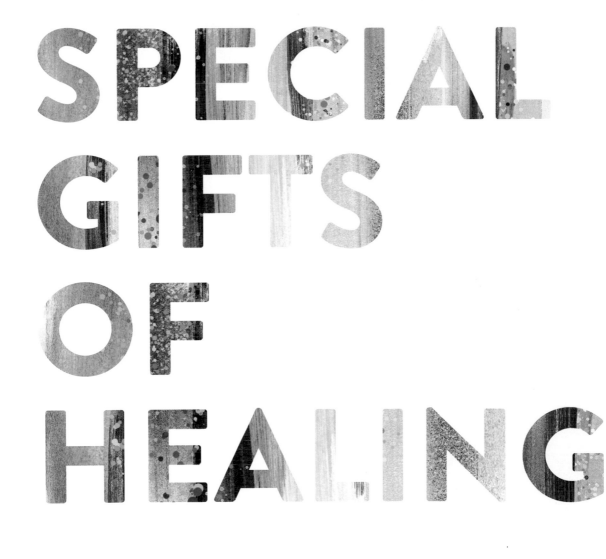

SPECIAL
GIFTS
OF
HEALING

IN FEW OTHER PROFESSIONS
ARE WE PRESENT AT LIFE'S
most momentous events,
FROM BIRTH TO DEATH,
FROM CRISIS TO RECOVERY.

DIANE BARNET

TO KNOW EVEN ONE LIFE
HAS BREATHED EASIER
because you have lived;
THAT IS TO
HAVE SUCCEEDED.

RALPH WALDO EMERSON

A nurse
WILL ALWAYS
GIVE US HOPE,
an angel
WITH A
STETHOSCOPE.

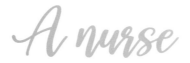

CARRIE LATET

Save one life
AND YOU'RE A HERO;
save 100 lives
AND YOU'RE A
HEALTH-CARE
WORKER.

♥

UNKNOWN

THE NURSE IS TEMPORARILY
THE CONSCIOUSNESS
OF THE UNCONSCIOUS,
THE LOVE OF LIFE
FOR THE SUICIDAL,
THE LEG OF THE AMPUTEE,
THE EYES OF THE NEWLY BLIND,
A MEANS OF LOCOMOTION
FOR THE INFANT,
THE KNOWLEDGE AND CONFIDENCE
OF THE YOUNG MOTHER,
AND A VOICE FOR THOSE
TOO WEAK TO SPEAK.

VIRGINIA HENDERSON

Love cures people—
BOTH THE ONES
WHO GIVE IT
AND THE ONES
WHO RECEIVE IT.

KARL MENNINGER

YOU'RE GOING TO BE THERE
WHEN A LOT OF PEOPLE
ARE BORN, AND WHEN
A LOT OF PEOPLE DIE.
IN MOST EVERY CULTURE,
SUCH MOMENTS ARE
REGARDED AS SACRED....
What an honor that is.

THOM DICK

NOT ALL ANGELS HAVE WINGS...
some have scrubs.

♥

UNKNOWN

IT WOULD
NOT BE POSSIBLE
to praise nurses
TOO HIGHLY.

♥

STEPHEN AMBROSE

THE PLANET DOES NOT NEED
MORE SUCCESSFUL PEOPLE.
The planet desperately needs
MORE PEACEMAKERS,
HEALERS, RESTORERS,
STORYTELLERS, AND
LOVERS OF ALL KINDS.

♥

DALAI LAMA

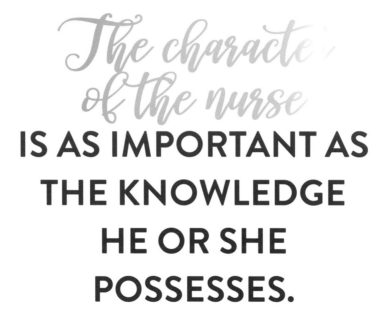

The character of the nurse

IS AS IMPORTANT AS
THE KNOWLEDGE
HE OR SHE
POSSESSES.

CAROLYN JARVIS

THE PHYSICIAN MUST NOT ONLY BE *the healer,* BUT OFTEN *the consoler.*

HARRIOT KEZIA HUNT

TO DO WHAT NOBODY ELSE WILL DO, IN A WAY THAT NOBODY ELSE CAN, IN SPITE OF ALL WE GO THROUGH IS *to be a nurse.*

RAWSI WILLIAMS

HEALTH-CARE WORKERS

are patient people.

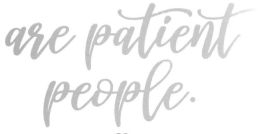

UNKNOWN

IT FEELS GOOD TO
HEAR SOMEONE SAY,
"Take care."
BUT IT FEELS
SO MUCH BETTER TO
HEAR SOMEONE SAY,
"I will take care of you."

UNKNOWN

WE ARE
FULLY AWARE OF
HOW PRECIOUS
each moment of life is.

PATRICIA BRATIANU

I SHARE IN THE JOY OF
NEWLY BORN BABIES AND
MIRACULOUSLY CURED DISEASES.
I SHARE IN THE HEARTBREAK OF
A CHILD TAKEN TOO SOON,
A DISEASE TOO POWERFUL,
A LIFE CHANGED FOREVER.
MY PATIENT IS OFTEN
AN ENTIRE FAMILY.

KATERI ALLARD

Our job...
IS TO CUSHION
THE SORROW
AND CELEBRATE
THE JOY EVERY DAY,
WHILE WE ARE
JUST DOING OUR JOBS.

♥

CHRISTINE BELLE

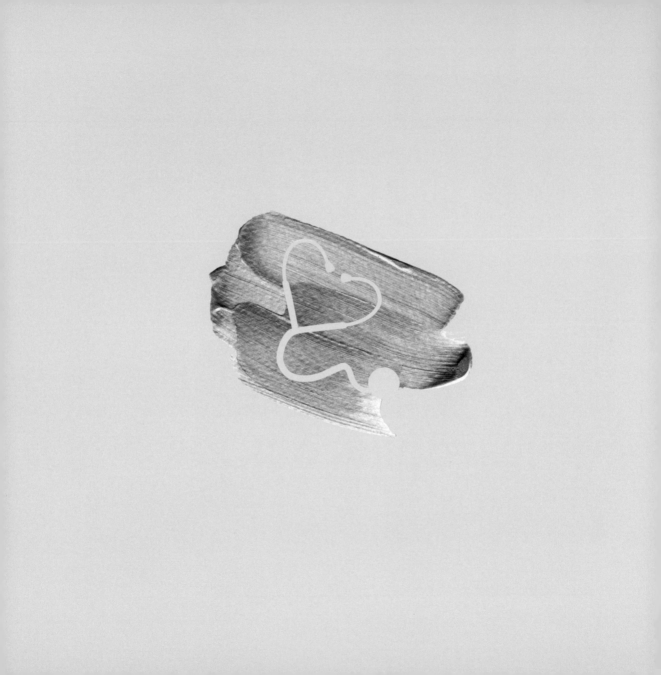

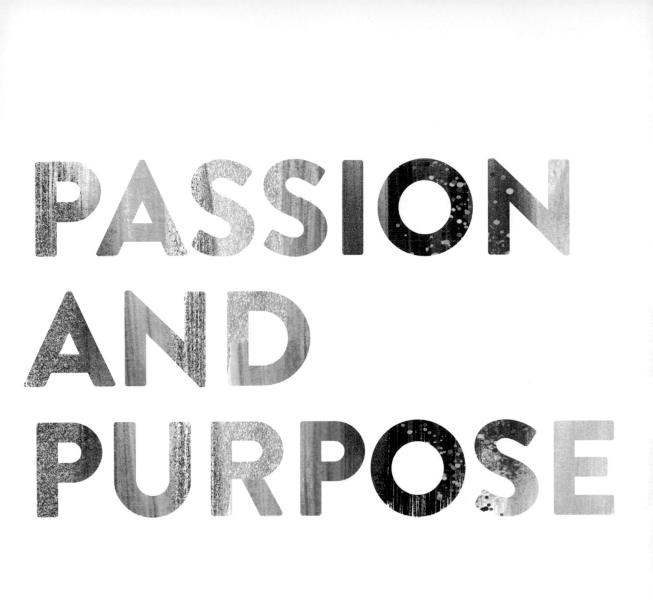

IT TAKES A VERY STRONG,
INTELLIGENT, AND
COMPASSIONATE PERSON
TO TAKE ON THE ILLS OF
THE WORLD WITH PASSION
AND PURPOSE AND WORK TO
MAINTAIN THE HEALTH AND
WELL-BEING OF THE PLANET.
NO WONDER WE'RE EXHAUSTED
AT THE END OF THE DAY!

DONNA WILK CARDILLO

A hero
IS SOMEONE WHO HAS
GIVEN HIS OR HER LIFE
TO SOMETHING BIGGER
THAN ONESELF.

JOSEPH CAMPBELL

WE MAKE A LIVING
by what we get,
BUT WE MAKE A LIFE
by what we give.

NORMAN MacEWEN

I ATTRIBUTE
MY SUCCESS TO THIS:
I NEVER GAVE
NOR TOOK

any excuse.

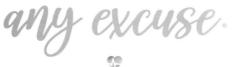

FLORENCE NIGHTINGALE

THE BEST WAY
to find yourself
IS TO LOSE YOURSELF
IN THE SERVICE
OF OTHERS.

MAHATMA GANDHI

Every nurse
WAS DRAWN TO NURSING BECAUSE OF A DESIRE TO CARE, TO SERVE, OR TO HELP.

CHRISTINA FEIST-HEILMEIER

IF WE DO NOT LAY OUT OURSELVES IN THE SERVICE OF MANKIND,

whom should we serve?

JOHN ADAMS

WHEN LOVE AND SKILL WORK TOGETHER,

expect a masterpiece.

♥

JOHN RUSKIN

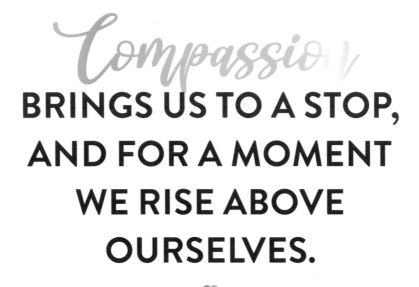

Compassion
BRINGS US TO A STOP,
AND FOR A MOMENT
WE RISE ABOVE
OURSELVES.

MASON COOLEY

THE PROFESSION
IS ALL ABOUT GRACE.
Helping people
IS A NOBLE CALLING.

KATHERINE SOH

WHEN A PERSON DECIDES
to become a nurse,
THEY MAKE THE MOST
IMPORTANT DECISION
OF THEIR LIVES.
THEY CHOOSE TO
DEDICATE THEMSELVES
TO THE CARE OF OTHERS.

MARGARET HARVEY

WHERE THE NEEDS
OF THE WORLD AND
YOUR TALENTS CROSS,
there lies your vocation.

ARISTOTLE

ONE OF THE
deep secrets of life
IS THAT ALL THAT IS
REALLY WORTH DOING
IS WHAT WE DO
FOR OTHERS.

LEWIS CARROLL

Nursing is the opposite of despair;

IT OFFERS THE OPPORTUNITY TO DO SOMETHING ABOUT SUFFERING.

TILDA SHALOF

The purpose of life is TO DISCOVER YOUR GIFT. *The work of life is* TO DEVELOP IT. *The meaning of life is* TO GIVE YOUR GIFT AWAY.

DAVID VISCOTT

I was born to be a nurse:
TO HOLD, TO AID,
TO SAVE, TO HELP,
TO TEACH, TO INSPIRE.
IT'S WHO I AM.
MY CALLING,
MY PASSION, MY LIFE,
AND MY WORLD.

♥

UNKNOWN

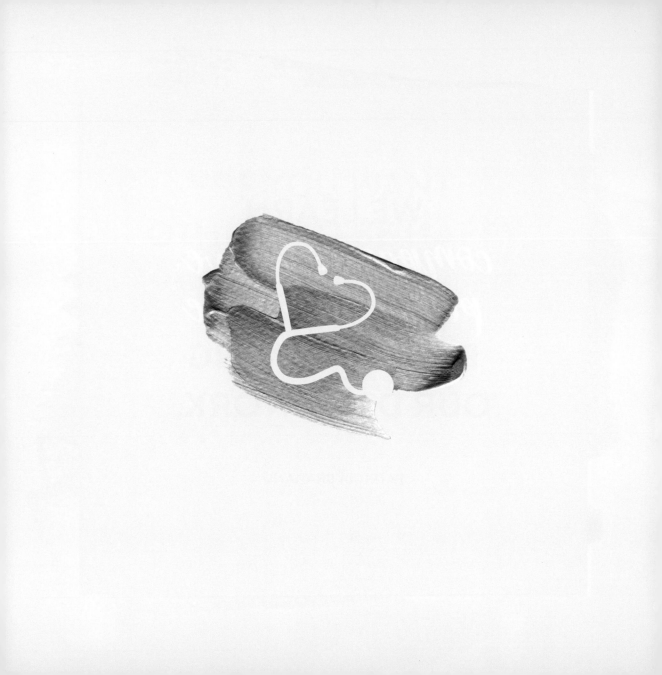

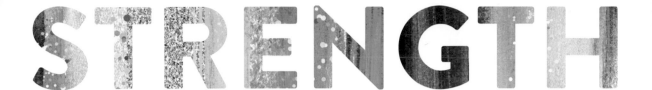
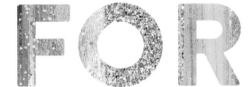
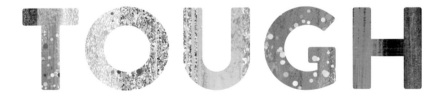
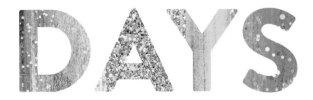

STRENGTH FOR TOUGH DAYS

I AM ONLY ONE,
BUT STILL I AM ONE.
I CANNOT DO EVERYTHING,
BUT STILL I CAN DO SOMETHING,
AND BECAUSE I CANNOT
DO EVERYTHING,
I WILL NOT REFUSE TO DO
SOMETHING THAT I CAN DO.

EDWARD EVERETT HALE

I MAY BE COMPELLED TO FACE DANGER,
but never fear it.

CLARA BARTON

YOU GAIN STRENGTH,
COURAGE, AND CONFIDENCE
BY EVERY EXPERIENCE
IN WHICH YOU REALLY STOP
TO LOOK FEAR IN THE FACE.
YOU MUST DO THE
THINGS WHICH YOU THINK
YOU CANNOT DO.

ELEANOR ROOSEVELT

NURSES ARE THERE WHEN
THE LAST BREATH IS TAKEN,
AND NURSES ARE THERE WHEN
THE FIRST BREATH IS TAKEN.
ALTHOUGH IT IS MORE
ENJOYABLE TO
CELEBRATE THE BIRTH,
IT IS JUST AS IMPORTANT
TO COMFORT IN DEATH.

CHRISTINE BELLE

CARING ABOUT OTHERS,
RUNNING THE RISK
OF FEELING,
AND LEAVING AN
IMPACT ON PEOPLE
brings happiness.

HAROLD KUSHNER

You treat a disease,
YOU WIN, YOU LOSE.
You treat a person,
I GUARANTEE YOU,
YOU'LL WIN,
NO MATTER WHAT
THE OUTCOME.

PATCH ADAMS

MOST OF THE IMPORTANT
THINGS IN THE WORLD
HAVE BEEN ACCOMPLISHED
BY PEOPLE WHO
HAVE KEPT ON TRYING
WHEN THERE SEEMED
TO BE NO HOPE AT ALL.

DALE CARNEGIE

ONLY IN
THE DARKNESS
CAN YOU

see the stars.

♥

MARTIN LUTHER KING, JR.

NEVER BELIEVE THAT
a few caring people
CAN'T CHANGE
THE WORLD.
FOR, INDEED,
THAT'S ALL
WHO EVER HAVE.

MARGARET MEAD

WHEN YOU'RE A NURSE
YOU KNOW THAT
EVERY DAY
you will touch a life
OR A LIFE
WILL TOUCH YOURS.

♥

UNKNOWN

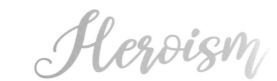

Heroism
**DOESN'T ALWAYS HAPPEN
IN A BURST OF GLORY.**
SOMETIMES
SMALL TRIUMPHS
AND LARGE HEARTS
**CHANGE THE COURSE
OF HISTORY.**

MARY ROACH

Courage is contagious.
EVERY TIME
WE CHOOSE COURAGE,
WE MAKE EVERYONE
AROUND US A LITTLE BETTER
AND THE WORLD
A LITTLE BRAVER.

BRENÉ BROWN

THOUSANDS OF CANDLES CAN BE LIGHTED FROM A *single candle.*

BUDDHA

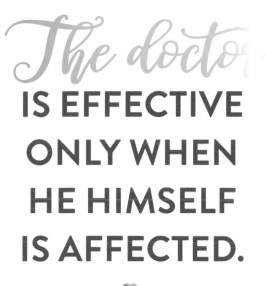

The doctor
IS EFFECTIVE
ONLY WHEN
HE HIMSELF
IS AFFECTED.

CARL JUNG

THERE ARE TWO WAYS
TO LIVE YOUR LIFE.
ONE IS AS THOUGH
NOTHING IS A MIRACLE.
THE OTHER IS AS IF
everything is.

ALBERT EINSTEIN

NURSES ARE
CONSTANTLY REMINDED
OF THE NECESSITY OF
VALUING THE DIGNITY AND
WORTH OF EVERY PERSON.
AS A RESULT, WE BECOME
BETTER PEOPLE.
Our souls are healed.

PATRICIA BRATIANU

SOME DAYS THERE WON'T BE A SONG IN YOUR HEART.

Sing anyway.

❤

EMORY AUSTIN

THE MOST IMPORTANT PART
OF OUR WORK IS ABOUT
MORE THAN OUTCOMES—
IT'S ABOUT THOSE MOMENTS
WHEN THE PATIENT, FAMILY,
AND CARE TEAM
ARE ALL WORKING
TOGETHER SEAMLESSLY,
dedicated to healing.

ERIKA KIMBALL

LET ME DEDICATE MY LIFE
TODAY TO THE CARE OF THOSE
WHO COME MY WAY.
LET ME TOUCH EACH ONE WITH
A HEALING HAND AND THE
GENTLE ART FOR WHICH I STAND.
AND THEN TONIGHT WHEN
THE DAY IS DONE, LET ME REST IN
PEACE IF I'VE HELPED JUST ONE.

UNKNOWN

I EXPECT TO PASS THROUGH
THIS WORLD BUT ONCE.
ANY GOOD, THEREFORE,
THAT I CAN DO OR
ANY KINDNESS I CAN SHOW
TO ANY FELLOW CREATURE,
let me do it now.

♥

STEPHEN GRELLET

AT THE
END OF THE DAY,
love and compassion
WILL WIN.

TERRY WAITE